# Medical Emergencies in Early Childhood and School-Age Settings, Revised Edition

---

## Emergency Telephone Numbers

**Emergency Medical Services (EMS):** _____

**Poison Control Center:**  <u>800-222-1222</u>_____

**Police Department:** _____

**Fire Department:** _____

**Health Consultant:** _____

**Physician:** _____

**Dentist:** _____

**Hospital:** _____

**Other:** _____

**When in doubt of whom to call, dial 911.**

---

In most communities, dialing 911 will access local emergency services. However, some communities do not have 911 access, and some cellular phone services do not automatically access the closest emergency services. The direct phone numbers for your local emergency services should be posted by the phone. For more information and recommendations about partnering with local emergency services, check out *Disaster Planning and Preparedness in Early Childhood and Schoolage Care Settings* (Redleaf Press 2014).

All teachers and staff members should be familiar with the Emergency Medical Services (EMS) in their community *before* they are actually needed for an emergency. Find out the answers to the following questions:

- What is the best telephone number to reach EMS?
- How fast will emergency help arrive?
- What hospital do they use? How long will it take to transport a child to the hospital?
- What authorization or documentation is required for them to treat and/or transport a child?
- May a staff member accompany the child to the hospital?

Familiarize children with emergency personnel and other community helpers as part of your curriculum. For curriculum suggestions and children's learning activities, check out *Growing, Growing Strong: A Whole Health Curriculum for Young Children* (Redleaf Press, 2014).

Redleaf *Quick* Guide

# Medical Emergencies

## IN EARLY CHILDHOOD AND SCHOOL-AGE SETTINGS

### Revised Edition

**Charlotte M. Hendricks, PhD**

Redleaf Press®
www.redleafpress.org
800-423-8309

Published by Redleaf Press
10 Yorkton Court
St. Paul, MN 55117
www.redleafpress.org

*Medical Emergencies in Early Childhood and School-Age Settings* is not a substitute for professional emergency medical care. Rather, its purpose it to help child care providers respond to medical emergencies and take appropriate action to maintain healthy, safe, and nurturing environments for children. Pediatric first aid and CPR training is recommended for all child care professionals.

First edition published 2008. Revised edition 2016.
Cover and interior design by Jim Handrigan
Interior typeset by Douglas Schmitz
Interior illustrations by Brian Trotter
Printed in the United States of America

Library of Congress Cataloging-in-Publication Data

Names: Hendricks, Charlotte Mitchell, 1957- , author.
Title: Medical emergencies in early childhood settings / Charlotte M.
   Hendricks.
Other titles: Redleaf quick guide.
Description: Revised edition. | St. Paul, MN : Redleaf Press, 2016. | Series:
   Redleaf quick guide | Includes bibliographical references.
Identifiers: LCCN 2015040967 | ISBN 9781605544373 (pbk. : alk. paper)
Subjects: | MESH: Child—Handbooks. | Emergencies—Handbooks. | Emergency
   Treatment—methods—Handbooks.
Classification: LCC RJ370 | NLM WS 39 | DDC 618.92/0025--dc23
LC record available at http://lccn.loc.gov/2015040967

Printed on acid-free paper                                              U22-06

# Contents

# Foreword

*Dr. Donald Palmer*

This book is written for you, the teacher. Its purpose is to provide you with a quick and accurate reference for appropriate action during medical emergencies occurring in early care and education (ECE) and school-age settings. Take some time to familiarize yourself with the information in and organization of this book so you can use it effectively if needed during an emergency situation.

First aid is the immediate care given to a person who has been injured or suddenly becomes ill, in order to stabilize and possibly address the situation until medical help is obtained as indicated. First aid in ECE and school-age settings may involve something as simple as washing and bandaging a scratched knee, or it may mean performing abdominal thrusts to clear a blocked airway.

All staff members who are involved in providing direct care for children should have training in pediatric first aid, including management of a blocked airway and administration of cardiopulmonary resuscitation (CPR).

The provision of first aid should be thoughtful, orderly, and rapid. During an emergency, first evaluate the situation. Find out what happened and who is involved. Quickly inspect the child who is injured or ill with a "hands off" approach (without touching the child). Evaluate the child's CABs: **C**hest compressions, **A**irway, and **B**reaths. You should complete the CABs in 10 seconds or less.

After this brief appraisal, be sure noninvolved children are adequately supervised and out of the way.

Quickly return to the child to perform a "hands on" evaluation. Does Emergency Medical Services (EMS) need to be called? What first aid actions can you give?

After these steps are completed, notify the child's parent or guardian. Comfort the ill or injured child, explain what has happened, and answer questions. Write a thorough incident report and determine if your licensing or regulatory agency needs to be notified.

Remember that prevention is the first, best form of treatment.

*Dr. Palmer is nationally recognized for his expertise and efforts to promote child health. Some of his accomplishments include being a member of the American Academy of Pediatrics (AAP) Committee on Early Childhood, Adoption, and Dependent Care; a reviewer of Caring for Our Children; a member of the steering committee for Pediatric First Aid for Caregivers and Teachers; a certified playground inspector; a member of the AAP Committee on Injury, Violence, and Poison Prevention; and the former president of the Alabama Chapter of AAP.*

# Standard Precautions

Most medical emergency situations in ECE and school-age settings are not life-threatening. These situations allow you time to wash your hands, put on gloves, and access first aid supplies. By following simple practices known as "standard precautions," you can help reduce the spread of infection and prevent transmission of blood-borne germs such as those that cause HIV/AIDS or hepatitis B.

Follow standard precautions in all medical emergencies or situations involving first aid or medical care. These procedures will help protect you, the injured or ill child, and other children and adults in the environment. The basics of standard precautions are:

- Wash hands with soap and running water.
- Wear nonporous, disposable, non-latex gloves.
- Carefully clean up spills that may contain blood or other body fluids.
- Clean contaminated surfaces.
- Sanitize or disinfect contaminated surfaces.
- Properly discard used gloves, bandages, tissues, and other items.
- Wash hands again after removing gloves.

## Hand Washing

Wash hands with liquid soap and running water. Lather well, then rub hands for **at least** 20 seconds. Clean the wrists, palms, fingers, in between fingers, back of hands, and around fingernails.

Liquid hand sanitizers (waterless soaps) and premoistened wipes **are not** an effective substitute for soap and running water. However, if soap and running water are not available (when transporting children or during nature walks, for example) the first aid responder should remove dirt from her hands with the wipes, and then apply liquid sanitizer (at least 60% alcohol) using the following procedure.

- Apply a generous amount of hand sanitizer into the palm of one hand.
- Rub hands together until sanitizer covers fingers, palms, and wrists. Hands should be completely covered.
- Let sanitizer air-dry.

## Non-latex Gloves

- Maintain an ample supply of single-use, nonporous, disposable gloves. Use non-latex gloves to avoid possible allergic reaction. Gloves should be powder-free.
- Gloves must be available **at all times** when children are present.

- Gloves must be discarded after one use.
- Hands must be washed **before** putting on gloves, and again **after** gloves are removed.

## Cleaning and Sanitizing

*Cleaning* removes visible spills, dirt, and debris. Clean all surfaces, including outdoor surfaces that are possibly contaminated with blood or other body fluids (including vomit, urine, stool, mucus, and saliva).

- Wear nonporous gloves.
- Clean up spills using paper towels, tissues, or rags. Use disposables if possible.
- Put soiled towels or rags into a plastic-lined receptacle for disposal or to launder/ sanitize later. Immediately tie bag shut and empty receptacle.
- Use soapy water to clean all surfaces.
- Rinse the surface with water.
- Sanitize surface.

*Sanitizing* means to reduce germs on surfaces to levels considered safe by public health code. *Disinfecting* means to destroy or kill most germs on surfaces. A mild bleach solution is an effective and inexpensive sanitizer/disinfectant.

- Mix fresh bleach solution each day. Old solution cannot kill germs.
- Use "regular" bleach products; avoid scented or "splashless" bleach products. It is recommended that only EPA-registered products be used. Follow the manufacturer's instructions when preparing bleach solution.
- Store undiluted bleach in a locked cabinet. Keep bleach solution out of children's reach.

### TO SANITIZE OR DISINFECT SURFACES:

- Wear nonporous gloves.
- Clean visible dirt and spills from the surface.
- Apply appropriate sanitizing or disinfecting solution to surfaces.
- Wet surface thoroughly with the solution and let air-dry.
- If surface must be wiped dry, allow solution to remain wet on surface for the amount of time recommended by the manufacturer.
- Properly dispose of towel or cloth used to wipe surface.
- Store sanitizing/disinfecting solution out of children's reach.
- Remove gloves and wash hands.

# Planning and Preparation

## Staff Training

All teachers should have training regarding medical emergencies.

- At least one teacher who is currently certified in pediatric first aid (including cardiopulmonary resuscitation [CPR]) must be available on site at all times and in all places where children are present.
- All teachers, substitute teachers, and volunteers involved in providing direct care for children should have up-to-date training in the following areas:
  - » Pediatric first aid, including management of a blocked airway (choking) and CPR
  - » Sanitation and standard precautions
  - » Child safety and injury prevention
- At least one teacher who is currently certified in pediatric CPR must be immediately available when children are involved in swimming and wading.
- At least one teacher who is currently certified in pediatric CPR must be immediately available when a child is known to have a specific special health need (such as cardiac arrhythmia) that makes the child more likely than a typical child to require cardiac resuscitation.
- Teachers and staff directly responsible for children with special health care needs should be trained in administration of all medical procedures and/or medications that might be required for that child (such as an epinephrine auto-injector or asthma inhaler). Training should be provided by a qualified health care professional.
- Program directors should regularly review teachers' ability to perform first aid and to respond to medical emergencies.
- Fully stocked first aid kits and children's life-sustaining medicines (such as epinephrine auto-injectors) must be clearly marked and immediately available to the teacher at all times, including on trips outside the facility.
- Teachers should have immediate access to communication (such as cellular phones) at all times and in all places where children are in care.

## Authorization and Documentation

Maintain current information on each child. Update the following information regularly according to your state licensing regulations:

- Names of parents, guardians, or other people who can authorize medical treatment
- Signed authorization forms, including all forms required under HIPAA (Health Insurance Portability and Accountability Act), such as Release of Information forms
- Names of family members and other emergency contacts and current phone numbers

- Names and phone numbers of each child's physician, dentist, and preferred hospital
- List of any allergies
- Diagnosis and treatment, including emergency care plan, for children with special health care needs, including specific indications for use and dose for any medications

Document all instances of illness or injury, no matter how minor, and the treatment provided. Provide specific details for every event. In some cases, medical emergencies must be reported to state licensing or other regulatory agencies.

## First Aid Kit

A first aid kit should be readily available wherever children are in care, including during field trips, when playing outdoors, and while being transported.

- First aid supplies must be stored in a clearly marked, closed container.
- A first aid kit must be accessible to teachers but locked or otherwise inaccessible to children.
- Restock the kit after each use.
- Include a checklist of items inside the kit. Check and document inventory monthly; replace missing, expired, or unusable items.
- **Do not** include medications in the kit unless prescribed for a specific child (such as an epinephrine auto-injector).
- Do not leave the kit in a vehicle or in direct heat.

**THE FIRST AID KIT SHOULD CONTAIN AT LEAST THE FOLLOWING ITEMS:**
- Disposable, nonporous, non-latex gloves
- Liquid soap
- Premoistened cloths and hand sanitizer of at least 60% alcohol (if water is not available to wash hands)
- Tissues
- Bandage scissors
- Tweezers
- Ear, forehead, or other non-glass digital thermometer (with instructions)
- Adhesive strip bandages (assorted sizes)
- Sterile gauze pads
- Flexible roller gauze
- Bandage tape
- Eye patch or dressing
- Safety pins
- Eye shield
- Triangular bandages
- Any prescribed emergency medication needed for a specific child (such as an epinephrine auto-injector or insulin)
- Sterile water

- Plastic zipper bags (assorted sizes) to make cold packs or dispose of used supplies
- Cold packs, either "instant" or put ice in a plastic bag and wrap in a cloth. Do not place ice or cold pack directly on a child's skin, because it can injure skin and tissue (frostnip).
- A copy of this Redleaf Quick Guide or a current standard first aid chart or first aid guide.
- Pen/pencil and notepad
- Cellular phone, radio, or other communication device
- Telephone numbers of Poison Control Center, paramedics, and other emergency services
- List of home, cellular, and work phone numbers for parents, family members, or emergency contact person for each child
- Flashlight
- Whistle

## ADDITIONAL ITEMS FOR FIRST AID SUPPLIES:

- Tooth preservation kit, such as Save-A-Tooth and EMT ToothSaver systems, which include a tooth container and fluid solution. This system can help preserve a tooth for longer times, increasing the possibility that the tooth can be saved.
- A bottle of sterile, nonpreserved ophthalmic saline solution can be included in the first aid kit and used to flush eyes. Solution is for one-time use only. Any unused solution must be disposed of and replaced with an unopened bottle.
- Activated charcoal is sometimes used after a poison has been ingested. It should be administered only with instruction from the Poison Control Center or a physician and ideally with parental knowledge and permission.

# Bleeding

Control of bleeding is a priority. Life-threatening amounts of blood can be lost very quickly.

- Determine where the blood is coming from, and whether bleeding has stopped.
  - » Call EMS (911) if bleeding is severe, appears to be arterial (bright red, spurting, or pulsing flow), or is not easily controlled within a few minutes.
  - » Some superficial wounds, such as those on the scalp, tend to bleed profusely but generally are not life-threatening.

## Controlling Bleeding

- Put on non-latex gloves.
- If possible, lay the child down. Comfort the child.
- Remove loose debris from the wound. **Do not** attempt to remove an object or glass imbedded in a wound, because it may cause more bleeding. Instead, place bandages around the object to secure object in place.
- Place gauze or other clean material on the wound.
- Apply direct pressure with your fingers or palm of your hand to the area that is bleeding. Continue pressure until the bleeding stops (usually 1 to 2 minutes). *See figure 1.*
- If blood soaks through, place additional gauze on top of the first compress. **Do not** remove the original compress.
- If no other injury (such as a fracture or head injury) is suspected, elevate the injured part of the body so it is above the level of the child's heart.
- Contact the child's family.

*figure 1*

### CALL EMS (911) IF:

- Bleeding is severe or appears to be arterial (bright red, spurting or pulsing flow).
- Bleeding does not stop with 5 minutes of continuous direct pressure. Continue to apply pressure until first responders arrive. **Do not** apply a tourniquet.
- The child is bleeding from the head.

- A body part is crushed, or partially or fully amputated.
  - » Keep the amputated body part clean.
  - » Wrap the body part with wet gauze using sterile water and place in a plastic bag. Place bag in ice water.
  - » Keep the body part *with the child.*
- An object is embedded deep within the wound.
- The child shows symptoms of **shock**. *See the section on Shock under "SUDDEN ILLNESS" for more information.*
- Internal injury or bleeding is suspected. Symptoms can include the following:
  - » The child complains of severe pain.
  - » The child appears very ill (pale, weak, clammy, fainting).
  - » Soft tissues (such as in the abdomen) are tender, swollen, or hard.
  - » The child has a rapid, weak pulse.
  - » The child has nausea or vomiting, or is vomiting blood.
  - » The child has bruising extending from the injured area.

Contact the child's family after EMS (911) has been called.

# Nosebleed

- Put on non-latex gloves.
- Help the child sit up with head tilted slightly forward. *See figure 2.*
- Pinch the nose closed. Apply gentle pressure for at least 5 minutes and up to 10 minutes.
- If possible, apply a cloth-wrapped cold pack to the child's nose and cheeks while holding the nose closed.
- Gently release the nose. If bleeding starts again, reapply the pressure for up to another 10 minutes.
- After the nosebleed stops, gently clean blood from the child's face and skin; provide clean clothing if necessary.
- Place all contaminated clothing in plastic sealed bags for parent pickup.
- Dispose of all bloody tissues and cloth in sealed plastic bags.
- Discourage the child from blowing or picking his nose.
- Have the child remain quiet for at least 30 minutes.

figure 2

**CALL EMS (911) IF:**
- The nosebleed cannot easily be controlled after 15 minutes.
- The child also feels dizzy or weak.
- It occurs after a blow to the head or a fall.
- The child is bleeding from other areas, such as gums.

Contact the child's family if EMS (911) has been called.

- Document the nosebleed and treatment; inform the child's family.

# Wounds, Cuts, and Blisters

## Open Wounds

- Put on non-latex gloves.
- Control the bleeding with direct pressure. *See "BLEEDING" for more information.*
- Contact the child's family and recommend picking up their child for **immediate medical attention** if the wound:
  - » Does not stop bleeding after 5 minutes or more of direct pressure.
  - » Appears deep.
  - » Will not stay closed by itself or if a cut or wound is longer than ½ inch.
  - » Is on the face or involves the eyes or ears.
  - » Is on the lip and crosses onto the cheek.
  - » Is from a bite (animal or human). *See "BITES AND STINGS" for more information.*
- For minor wounds (cuts, scratches, and scrapes), once the bleeding stops, gently wash the wound with soap and water, then apply a clean dressing and bandage.

## Puncture Wounds

Puncture wounds may be deep (such as a knife wound) or shallow (such as a splinter). These wounds generally do not bleed much; however, puncture wounds can be serious.

- Put on non-latex gloves.
- If the object is small and can be easily removed (such as a nail or thumbtack that has been stepped on), then remove the object.
- Allow the wound to bleed freely for a few minutes to help remove debris.
- After a few minutes, control bleeding with direct pressure. *See "BLEEDING" for more information.*
- Once bleeding stops, gently wash the wound with soap and water.
- Apply a clean dressing and bandage.
- Contact the child's family and recommend they consult their doctor's office for further instruction and to confirm tetanus booster status.

*figure 3*

**CALL EMS (911) IF:**

- The penetrating object is large or deeply embedded (such as glass, a stick, or a knife).
  - » **Do not** remove objects that are protruding (sticking out). Removal could cause further internal damage and severe bleeding.
  - » Hold the child still and immobilize the object. Place bandages around the object to secure object in place or hold the object still until first responders arrive. *See figure 3.*

Contact child's family.

## Splinters/Slivers

If the splinter is small and is sticking out of the skin, it probably can be easily removed. If possible, splinter/sliver removal is best left to a parent or health care professional.

- Clean tweezers with soap and water.
- Put on non-latex gloves.
- Grasp the splinter with tweezers. Gently pull the splinter so it comes out from the same direction that it went into the skin.
- **Do not** use a needle or other invasive procedure to remove splinters.
- After the splinter is removed, gently wash the wound with soap and water.
- Apply a clean dressing and bandage, if needed.
- Inform the child's family that you removed a splinter.

If the splinter is large or deeply embedded, or if you cannot easily remove the entire splinter with clean tweezers, then seek medical attention.

## Stickers

Stickers, such as spines from a caterpillar or cactus stickers, may be removed with sticky tape.

## Blisters

- Put on non-latex gloves.
- Protect blisters with a clean bandage. **Do not** break blisters.
- Contact the child's family and recommend medical attention if the blister is large (such as larger than the size of a quarter) or if there are multiple blisters.

### PRESCRIPTION FOR PREVENTION

- Check outdoor play areas each day and remove trash, sticks, glass, or other debris.
- Regularly inspect wooden play equipment for splinters; repair as needed.

# CPR

> ## Call EMS (911) if a child shows any problems with breathing.
>
> ## A child who is not breathing can sustain brain damage or die very quickly.

**START CPR WHEN A CHILD IS:**

- not breathing
- does not have a pulse
- is unconscious

**CHECK FOR RESPONSIVENESS. TAP THE INFANT'S FOOT, OR RUB THE CHILD, AND SHOUT, "ARE YOU OKAY?"**

- If a child is not responsive when found
  » Provide five cycles (about two minutes) of lifesaving CPR (30 compressions and 2 breaths), before leaving child to call EMS (911).
  » Check for breathing.
  » Call EMS (911).
  » If an AED is available, turn it on and follow instructions for use.

- If a child becomes non-responsive in your care
  » Shout for help. Call EMS (911).
  » Check for breathing.
  » Provide five cycles (about two minutes) of lifesaving CPR (30 compressions and 2 breaths).
  » If an AED is available, turn it on and follow instructions for use.

**IF THE CHILD IS *NOT* BREATHING, BEGIN CPR.**

Remember the sequence of C-A-B

**C—Compressions**: Chest compressions performed properly compress the heart, pumping blood and oxygen throughout the body until the heart resumes beating.

**A—Airway**: Open the airway for effective breathing.

**B—Breathing**: Breathing pushes air into the child's lungs. Use gentle breaths, forcing air into lungs can cause damage.

## C—Begin Chest Compressions

- Place the child on his back on a firm, flat surface. Give 30 chest compressions. Compressions should be FAST with no pausing. Count the 30 compressions quickly: "1-2-3-4-5-6-7-8-9-10-11-12-13-14-15-16-17-18-19-20-21-22-23-24-25-26-27-28-29-30 off."
- Each time, let the chest rise completely.

### INFANTS:

- Place 2 fingers (index and middle fingers) on the infant's breastbone just below the nipple line, and above the bottom tip of the breastbone. Keep fingers on the breastbone; compressing only the breastbone. *See figure 4.*
- Give 30 chest compressions, pushing the breastbone down approximately ⅓ of the chest depth (about 1½ inches)

*figure 4*

### TODDLERS:

- Place the heel of your hand on the child's breastbone just below the nipple line, and above the bottom tip of the breastbone. Use one or two hands as appropriate for the size of the child. *See figure 5.*
- Give 30 chest compressions, pushing the breastbone down approximately ⅓ of the chest depth (about 2 inches)

*figure 5*

## A—Open the Airway

- Use the head-tilt/chin-lift method to open the child's airway. *See figure 6.*
  » Place your hand on the child's forehead. Tilt head back slightly.
  » Place fingers of your other hand under the child's chin. Lift gently.
- Look for breathing.
  » Look to see if the chest and abdomen are rising and falling with breaths.
  » Take 5 to 10 seconds to do this.

## B—Breathing

If there is no breathing, begin CPR.

*figure 6*

### INFANTS:

- Cover the infant's mouth and nose tightly with your mouth.
- Use a CPR breathing barrier if available. *See figure 7.*

**TODDLERS AND OLDER CHILDREN:**

- Pinch the nose shut and gently seal the child's mouth with your mouth.
- Give 2 slow breaths immediately following each other.
- Watch to see if the child's chest rises and falls. If chest does not rise and fall, reposition the child's head and/or jaw to open the airway, and repeat breaths.
- Allow the air to flow out of the chest between breaths.
- Repeat  CPR cycles of 30 compressions and 2 breaths.
- Continue CPR until the child begins breathing or EMS arrives.

*figure 7*

## Using an AED

- Turn on AED. Follow the voice and/or visual prompts.
- Wipe the child's bare chest dry.
- Attach pads. If pads risk touching each other, use front-to-back placement.
- Plug in connector, if necessary.
- Stand clear. Make sure no one, including you, is touching the child.
- Analyze heart rhythm. Push the "analyze" button, if necessary. Let AED analyze the heart rhythm.
- Deliver shock.
- Follow prompts on AED. If a shock is advised:
    - » Make sure no one, including you, is touching the child.
    - » Say, "Everyone, stand clear."
    - » Push the "shock" button, if necessary.
- After delivering the shock, or if no shock is advised:
    - » Perform 5 cycles of CPR.
    - » Continue to follow the prompts of the AED.

## PR℞ESCRIPTION FOR PREVENTION

- Train all teachers and staff in pediatric CPR.
- The directions for CPR breathing and chest compression are revised and updated often. It is wise to check the website of the American Heart Association (www.americanheart.org) or the American Red Cross (www.redcross.org) regularly to make sure you are familiar with the latest methods.

# Choking

- Observe child for symptoms of choking.
- Call EMS (911). If you are alone, provide 1 minute of lifesaving first aid care, and then call EMS (911).
- If the child is coughing:
  » Encourage coughing. It is the best way to remove a blockage.
  » **Do not** pat the child on the back.
  » **Do not** hold up the child's arms or hold child upside down.
- Look inside the child's mouth.
- If object is easy to remove with your fingers, carefully remove it.
  » **Do not** "finger sweep" the mouth to remove the object. You might push it in deeper.
- If the object is **not** removed and/or the child stops breathing, follow the procedures for "Infant Choking" and "Toddler or Older Child Choking" below.

## Infant Choking (1 year of age and younger)

If the infant is **responsive** (conscious) and not breathing:

- Administer a combination of 5 back blows and 5 chest thrusts.
- Back blows:
  » Lay the infant face down on your forearm, with the infant's feet up toward your shoulder.
  » Place your hand around the infant's jaw and neck for support.
  » Rest your arm against your thigh for support. Use the heel of your other hand to give 5 quick, sharp back blows between the infant's shoulder blades.
  » If the object does not fall out of the infant's mouth, give 5 chest thrusts.
- Chest thrusts: *See figure 8.*
  » Turn the infant chest up, resting on your forearm.
  » Support your arm against your thigh. The infant's head should be lower than your trunk.
  » Place 2 fingers (index and middle fingers) from your other hand on the infant's breastbone slightly below the nipple line, but above the bottom tip of the breastbone.
  » Give 5 chest thrusts in rapid succession, pushing the breastbone down approximately ½ to 1 inch.

*figure 8*

- Put on non-latex gloves and check inside the infant's mouth after you do the chest thrusts. If you see the object causing the choking, carefully remove it. Then observe the infant's breathing. If the infant is not breathing, begin CPR.
- If the object is not removed, continue alternating back blows, chest thrusts, and checking mouth until first responders arrive, or the object is removed, or the child becomes unresponsive.

If the infant is **not responsive** (becomes unconscious) and not breathing, begin CPR. *See "CPR" for more information.*

- Look for breathing.
- If the infant does not start to breathe after opening the airway:
  - » Begin 30 chest compressions.
  - » Check mouth. Remove the object only if it is visible.
  - » Repeat until the infant begins to breathe or first responders arrive.

## Toddler or Older Child Choking

- If the child is **responsive** (conscious) and not breathing:
- Administer abdominal thrusts.
  - » Stand or kneel behind the child. Pull the child close to you.
  - » Make a fist and place it just above the child's navel, and below the breastbone.
  - » Cover your fist with your other hand, and give a quick upward and inward thrust to the child's abdomen.
- Continue abdominal thrusts until first responders arrive, the object is removed, or the child becomes unresponsive.

If the child is **not responsive** (becomes unconscious) and not breathing, begin CPR. *See "CPR" for more information.*

- Check for responsiveness.
- Open the airway.
- Look for breathing.
- Put on non-latex gloves and look in mouth for an object. Remove it if possible.
- If the child does not start to breathe after opening the airway:
  - » Begin 30 chest compressions, pushing the breat-bone down approximately 1½ inches.
  - » Check mouth. Remove the object only if it is visible.
  - » Repeat until the child begins to breathe or first responders arrive.

## Strangulation or Suffocation

- Call EMS (911).
- Remove object (cord, pillow, plastic, soft mattress).
- Check breathing.
- If the child is not breathing, begin CPR.

---

### P℞ESCRIPTION FOR PREVENTION

- Avoid serving foods that are potential choking hazards, such as hot dogs, popcorn, hard pretzels, and hard candy.
- Empty all containers, such as wading pools or buckets, when not in use. Never leave standing water unattended.
- **Do not** allow latex balloons or plastic dry cleaning bags in the environment.

# Poisoning

> ## Poisons can affect the body quickly!
> ## CONTACT EMS (911) IMMEDIATELY!
> ### Call the Poison Control Center at 800-222-1222.

## Swallowed Poison

Many substances are toxic, especially for young children. Medications, alcoholic beverages, cleaning supplies, chemicals, cosmetics, mouthwash, and some plants are just a few of the toxic substances children may encounter.

- Call EMS (911).
- Put on non-latex gloves and remove traces of the poisonous substance from the child's mouth with a napkin or tissue. Check the mouth carefully, including the roof of the mouth, and remove what you can see. **Do not** "sweep" the back of the throat with your finger, as this could push the substance farther into the child's throat.
- While waiting for first responders to arrive, call the Poison Control Center at 800-222-1222. Have the following information available:
  » Child's age and weight
  » What was swallowed (have the container or plant with you to describe)
  » Amount swallowed
  » Time the substance was swallowed
  » Child's condition
- Follow instructions from the Poison Control Center.
- Contact the child's family after EMS (911) has been called.

Observe the child for breathing difficulties (shortness of breath, wheezing, coughing). If the child stops breathing, begin **CPR (30 compressions and 2 breaths)** while waiting for first responders to arrive. *See "CPR" for more information.*

- If the child vomits and becomes unresponsive or unconscious, place the child on his side to prevent choking.
- When first responders arrive:
  » Be prepared to provide detailed information regarding the poisoning situation.
  » Give them the product container or a piece of the plant swallowed.
  » If the child vomits, give first responders a sample of the vomit.

## Inhaled Poison

Poisoning from inhaled fumes, such as carbon monoxide, can be life-threatening. Poisoning can also occur by inhaling fumes from substances such as rubber cement, model glue, or petroleum products.

- Remove the child (and everyone else) from the toxic area. This may require evacuation from the building.
- Call EMS (911).
- While waiting for first responders to arrive, call the Poison Control Center at 800-222-1222. Have the following information available:
  » Child's age and weight
  » What was inhaled
  » Time the substance was inhaled
  » Child's condition
- Follow instructions from the Poison Control Center.
- Contact the child's family after EMS (911) has been called.

Observe the child for breathing difficulties (shortness of breath, wheezing, coughing). If the child stops breathing, begin CPR (30 compressions and 2 breaths) while waiting for first responders to arrive. *See "CPR" for more information.*

## Skin Contact (irritating chemicals or substances)

Some substances, such as cleaning chemicals, can cause skin irritation.

- Immediately and thoroughly wash the area with soap and running water.
- Call the Poison Control Center at 800-222-1222.
- Follow instructions from the Poison Control Center. **Do not** follow any emergency instructions printed on product labels. Labels may be out-of-date or have incorrect treatment information.
- If the skin appears burned or the child is in pain, call EMS (911). *See "BURNS" for more information on treating chemical burns.*
- Contact the child's family.

## Poison Ivy, Poison Oak, or Other Plants

Certain plants, such as poison ivy, poison oak, or sumac, can cause a rash or other reaction. If contact with one of these plants is suspected:

- Immediately and thoroughly wash the area with soap and running water.
- Contact the child's family and inform them of the possible exposure.

---

### PRESCRIPTION FOR PREVENTION

- Store all medications in locked cabinets, out of children's reach.
- Store potentially toxic substances, such as cleaning supplies, out of reach, out of sight, and in areas that are inaccessible to children.
- Inspect play areas and carefully remove potentially harmful or toxic plants or fungi (for example, mushrooms).

# Allergic Reactions

Children can have allergic reactions to almost any substance, including medications, latex, insect stings, pollen, mold, food, or environmental triggers such as smoke, perfumes, or aerosols. Most reactions are mild. However, severe allergic reactions can be life-threatening.

## Anaphylaxis (severe allergic reaction)

Anaphylaxis is a **life-threatening problem** caused by a severe allergic reaction to a substance, such as a food (for example, peanuts), medication, or an insect bite or sting. Symptoms can occur quickly or may not appear until **minutes or hours** after the exposure.

- Call EMS (911) if the child has been exposed to a food, insect sting, medication, or other substance that has triggered a severe reaction in the past.
- Call EMS (911) if you observe symptoms of serious reaction (anaphylaxis), such as:
  - » Rash or hives on the body
  - » Itching, including in the mouth
  - » Swelling of the face, lips, tongue, or throat
  - » Swelling of the body part where the sting or bite occurred (more than just minor swelling of the skin where stung/bitten)
  - » Difficulty swallowing or speaking
  - » Dizziness, unexplained confusion, fainting, or loss of consciousness
  - » Breathing problems (shortness of breath, wheezing, coughing)
  - » Abdominal pain, nausea, vomiting, or other sudden illness
- Be prepared to administer CPR if necessary while waiting for first responders to arrive. *See "CPR" for more information.*
- A child who has had a previous severe reaction may have a doctor-prescribed auto-injector of epinephrine (such as **EpiPen Jr**). Injectable epinephrine should be administered only if prescribed for that child by a physician.

## Auto-Injector of Epinephrine (such as EpiPen Jr)

- Epinephrine should not be used unless prescribed by the child's physician.
- If prescribed, the auto-injector **must** be kept near the child at all times.
- Store the auto-injector at room temperature in a safe, dry place accessible to teachers but out of children's reach. Check expiration date frequently. **Note**: Do not store the auto-injector in a vehicle or other place where it can freeze or overheat.
- Teachers should be trained by medical personnel in correct use of the auto-injector.

To use an auto-injector:

- Hold the auto-injector in your hand and make a fist around it.
- Remove the safety cap.

- Place the orange tip of the injector near the fleshy part of the child's outer thigh. You can inject through the child's clothing. **Do not** inject into a vein or the buttocks.
- With a rapid motion, push the auto-injector firmly against the thigh and hold it in place until the medication is injected, about 10 seconds. *See figure 9.*
- Remove the auto-injector; replace it into the safety tube or other container.
- Call EMS (911).
- Give the auto-injector to first responders.
- Note: Follow directions on the prescribed epinephrine auto-injectors.

*figure 9*

## Mild Allergic Reactions

Mild allergic reactions may include redness of skin; itching, stuffy, or runny nose; sneezing; and itchy or watery eyes.

- If possible, remove the allergen or irritant.
  » If the trigger is environmental (such as perfume or smoke), remove the child from the area.
  » If the reaction is caused by skin contact with a substance, wash the child's skin with warm, soapy water.
- Observe the child for symptoms of serious allergic reaction. *See the Anaphylaxis section on the previous page for more information.*
- Refer to the child's medical record for information about previous allergic reactions.
  » If the child has a prescribed health care plan, follow those instructions.
  » Call EMS (911) if the child has been exposed to a food, insect sting, medication, or other substance that has triggered a severe reaction in the past.
  » A child who has had a previous severe reaction may have doctor-prescribed injectable epinephrine (such as EpiPen Jr). *See the Anaphylaxis section on the previous page for more information on injectable epinephrine.*
  » Contact the child's family and recommend medical attention.
  » Families should notify the child's doctor of any reaction, especially a reaction to medication. The next exposure to the substance could result in a more severe reaction.
- Continue to observe the child for symptoms of serious allergic reaction, including breathing problems or **shock.** *See the section on Shock under "SUDDEN ILLNESS" for more information.*

## PRᵪESCRIPTION FOR PREVENTION

- Document any allergies of children. Be sure all staff members are aware of potential allergy triggers.
- If a child is severely allergic to a substance such as peanuts, create a "peanut-safe" environment. This means products that contain peanuts or peanut byproducts are not allowed in the facility. Most serious food-allergic reactions are from peanuts, tree nuts, fish, and shellfish.
- Avoid use of aerosols, air fresheners, cleaners, perfumes, and tobacco products.

# Bites and Stings

## Animal Bite

- Control bleeding with direct pressure. *See "BLEEDING" for more information.*
- Wash the wound area with soap and water.
- If the **skin is broken**, contact the child's family and recommend immediate medical attention.
- If the **skin is not broken**, apply a cloth-wrapped cold pack to the bite area and comfort the child.
- Document all details of the incident, including the following information:
  » Description of the animal that bit the child
  » Location of the animal (including owner's name and address, if known)
  » Date of the animal's last rabies vaccination, if known
  » Any recent unusual behavior by the animal

### CALL EMS (911) IF:

- The child was bitten by a wild or stray animal; an animal whose rabies vaccination status is unknown; or an animal that is acting strangely.
- The child was bitten on the face, neck, or hand, or near a joint.
- The wound is deep.
- There are several bites.

## Human Bite

Infants and toddlers put their mouths on people and toys, and many toddlers try biting. Most bites are not medically serious. However, there is a risk of infection if the skin is broken.

- Step in between the children to prevent further biting. Stay calm; do not raise your voice.
- Help the child who was bitten before redirecting the other child.

If the **skin is broken**:

- Control bleeding (if any).
- Wash the wound with soap and water.
- Apply a cloth-wrapped cold pack to the bite area.
- Comfort the child.

- Contact the child's family.
- Recommend the child's family check with their health care provider about additional care.

If the **skin is not broken**:

- Apply a cloth-wrapped cold pack to the bite area.
- Comfort the child.

## Insect Bite or Sting

Most bites and stings cause mild reactions.

- Inspect the affected area. Remove any body parts of the stinging or biting insect that may remain on or in the child's skin.

figure 10

  » Remove a stinger by scraping it with a plastic card (such as a credit card). *See figure 10.* Gently scrape so it comes out from the same direction that it went into the skin. **Do not** use tweezers or squeeze the stinger.
  » Remove caterpillar spines from a child's skin with sticky tape.
- Wash the area with soap and water.
- Apply a cloth-wrapped cold pack to reduce pain and swelling.
- If the bite involves the limbs (arms, legs), keep the affected body part elevated. (Example: If the hand is stung, raise the child's hand/arm so it is higher than the level of the child's heart.)
- Observe the child for any symptoms of serious reaction. *See the section on Anaphylaxis under "ALLERGIC REACTIONS" for more information.* A child can have a serious reaction to a sting or to multiple stings, even if the child has had no previous allergic reaction.

## Spider Bite

Most spiders are venomous and cause mild reactions. However, bites from certain spiders can be serious and even life-threatening.

- Wash the bite area with soap and water.
- Apply a cloth-wrapped cold pack to reduce pain and swelling.
- Call the Poison Control Center at 800-222-1222 for further instruction.
- Contact the child's family and recommend medical attention.

Call EMS (911) if you suspect the bite is from a black widow or brown recluse spider. It will be helpful to first responders if you can describe the spider or if you can catch or kill the spider (without squashing it beyond recognition).

### Tick Bite

- Remove the tick as soon as you discover it.
- Use tweezers to grasp the tick near its head, close to the child's skin. *See figure 11.*
  - » Gently pull so the tick will come out from the same direction in which it entered the skin.
  - » Continue gentle pressure for several seconds, until the tick lets go.
  - » **Do not** twist or jerk the tick. **Do not** rupture the tick's body.
- Wash the bite area with soap and water.
- After removing the tick:
  - » Place the tick in a dry plastic bag or container for possible identification.
  - » Inform the child's family that you have removed a tick from the child.
  - » Ticks can carry life-threatening diseases such as Lyme disease and Rocky Mountain spotted fever. If a child has an embedded tick (the head is under the skin), strongly recommend that the child's family consult their health care provider for further instruction.

*figure 11*

### Scorpion Sting

Scorpion stings may cause localized pain that increases rapidly. The pain may travel up the limb (arm or leg) that was stung. A child may have a severe reaction, including breathing problems, paralysis, or tremors.

- Call EMS (911).
- Wash the sting area with soap and water.
- Apply a cloth-wrapped cold pack.
- Notify the child's family of the sting.
- Observe the child for signs of serious reaction. *See the section on Anaphylaxis under "ALLERGIC REACTIONS" for more information.*

## Snake Bite

- Call EMS (911).
- Wash the area with soap and water.
- Remove any potentially constricting items, such as jewelry, from the bitten area.
- Keep the child calm and the body part still. Keep the bitten area *lower* than the heart level.
- **Do not** apply an ice pack to a snake bite.
- Call the Poison Control Center at 800-222-1222 for advice. It will be helpful if you can describe the snake. However, **do not** try to catch the snake.
- Notify the child's family of the bite.
- Observe the child for signs of serious reaction. *See the section on Anaphylaxis under "ALLERGIC REACTIONS" for more information.*

## PRESCRIPTION FOR PREVENTION

- Enclose outdoor play areas with fencing; keep gates securely latched.
- Keep outdoor play areas clean and free of trash, garbage, or debris.
- Check outdoor play area and play equipment each day for insect nests, spiderwebs, and anthills.
- Trim bushes and shrubs off the ground and remove leaves and debris.

# Burns

## Thermal Burns (burns due to contact with a hot surface, hot liquid, or fire

- Run cool water over the burned skin.
- Continue to cool the skin with water until the pain stops or the child gets medical attention.
- Burns can cause swelling. Remove any potentially constricting items in the burn area, such as rings or bracelets, if they can be *easily* removed. **Do not** attempt to remove items if removal is difficult or may cause further injury to the skin and tissue.
- **Do not** attempt to remove clothing or jewelry that may be stuck to the burned skin.
- **Do not** apply butter, ointment, cream, or lotion to the burned area.

### CALL EMS (911) IF:

- The burn is on an infant or toddler.
- The burn involves the face, scalp, hands, feet, or genitals.
- The burn is large, deep, or forms blisters.
- The burn area is raw, ash white, black, leathery, or charred.
- Clothing or jewelry is stuck to the burned skin.
- The child shows symptoms of **shock**. *See the section on Shock under "SUDDEN ILLNESS" for more information.*

## Chemical Burns

- Brush any dry chemicals from the skin.
- Rinse the affected skin with cool running water.
- Call EMS (911).
- Continue to rinse the area until first responders arrive.
- Call the Poison Control Center at 800-222-1222. Have the following information available:
  » Child's age and weight
  » Chemical substance or ingredients (have the container with you to describe)
  » Area of body/skin affected
  » Amount of chemical
  » Time exposure occurred
  » Child's condition, including description of skin
- Follow instructions from the Poison Control Center. Do not follow any emergency instructions printed on product labels. Labels may be out-of-date or have incorrect treatment information.

- Remove contaminated clothing.
  - » Avoid spreading the chemical to other areas of the child's body. **Do not** remove a contaminated shirt by pulling it over the child's head.
  - » If necessary, carefully cut clothing to remove it easily.
  - » **Do not** attempt to remove clothing that is stuck to the child's skin.
- Remove any potentially constricting items in the burn area, such as rings or bracelets, if they can be easily removed. **Do not** attempt to remove items if removal is difficult or may cause further injury to the skin and tissue.
- If the chemical burned the eye, call EMS (911) and flush the eye gently with water for 15 minutes or until first responders arrive.

## Electrical Burns

- Remove the child from the electrical source.
  - » Turn off the power source *before* touching the child.
  - » If power cannot be turned off, push or pull the child away from the source with an object that does not conduct electricity (such as a wooden or plastic object or a thickly folded *dry* cloth).
- Call EMS (911).
- Check the child for breathing. If necessary, begin CPR. *See "CPR" for more information.*
- Observe child for symptoms of shock. *See the section on Shock under "SUDDEN ILLNESS" for more information.*

## PR${}_X$ESCRIPTION FOR PREVENTION

- Do not allow children access to hot appliances.
- Turn hot water thermostats to 120°F or lower.
- Cover all electrical outlets when not in use.
- Inspect and replace worn or frayed appliance cords.
- Teach children and practice "Stop, drop, and roll" to put out clothing that has caught on fire.

# Head, Neck, and Spine Injuries

Injury to the head, neck, or spine (back) requires **immediate** medical attention.

**CALL EMS (911) IF:**

- The injury resulted from a fall, a blow to the head or back, a vehicle crash, or another significant force.
- You observe or the child complains of any of the following symptoms as a result of a head, neck, or spine injury:
  - » Unconsciousness, even if only for a few seconds
  - » Bleeding from any part of the head
  - » Bleeding or fluid from the nose, ear, or mouth
  - » Unusual sleepiness or listlessness
  - » "Goose egg" or swelling, especially of an infant's fontanel ("soft spot")
  - » Pale, sweaty appearance
  - » Seizure
  - » Severe headache
  - » Neck pain or stiffness; pain radiating through the shoulders
  - » Vomiting
  - » Loss of bladder or bowel control
  - » Difficulty walking or moving arms or legs
  - » Dizziness, weakness, or paralysis
  - » Blurred vision
  - » Confusion or memory loss
  - » Slurred or difficult speech

Notify the child's family. After EMS (911) has been called. If EMS (911) is not called, notify the child's family and strongly encourage them to seek medical attention for further evaluations.

**IF SEVERE INJURY IS SUSPECTED:**

- **Do not** move the child while waiting for first responders to arrive unless the child is in immediate danger of further injury.
- Calm the child and encourage the child to remain still.
- Observe the child for breathing problems (shortness of breath, wheezing, coughing).
- If the child stops breathing and CPR is necessary, **avoid tilting or moving the head and neck.** *See "CPR" for more information.*

# Bone and Muscle Injuries

*(When head, neck, or spine injury is not suspected.)*

Bone and muscle injuries (sprain, strain, fracture, or dislocation) require medical attention.

- Stop the child's activity immediately.

**CALL EMS (911) IF:**

- There is obvious swelling of the injured joint or area.
- There is an abnormal shape or position of the area (for example, an arm or leg is at an unnatural angle or position).
- The suspected bone/muscle injury involves an open wound.
- The child complains of significant pain when the injured part is touched or moved.
- The child shows symptoms of shock. *See the section on Shock under "SUDDEN ILLNESS" for more information.*
    - » **Do not** move the injured part while waiting for first responders to arrive.
    - » **Do not** move the child (unless the child is in immediate danger of further injury).
    - » **Do not** encourage the child to move the injured body part.
    - » **Do not** attempt to "straighten" or "relocate" the injured limb or joint.
    - » **Do not** attempt to apply a splint or compression bandage. This level of treatment should be administered by a trained health care professional.
- Contact the child's family after EMS (911) has been called.

If the injury appears to be minor and EMS (911) is **not** called:

- Have the child sit or lie in a comfortable position.
- Help the child keep the injured part still if movement causes pain.
- Apply a cloth-wrapped cold pack for 20 minutes every hour.
- Elevate the injured part (if arm or leg) above the level of the heart by supporting on pillows or blankets.
- Contact the child's family and explain the nature of the injury. Recommend that the family seek medical attention for the child.

## P℞ESCRIPTION FOR PREVENTION

- Install approved resilient surfacing under and around all play equipment. *See "RESOURCES" for more information on the U.S. Consumer Product Safety Commission's Handbook for Public Playground Safety.*
- Require that each child wear a helmet when playing on wheeled toys.
- Install secure child-level handrails for all stairways. Install a nonslip surface on steps and ramps.
- Keep pathways clear. Provide adequate lighting.

# Heat-Related Conditions

## Heat Exhaustion

Heat exhaustion can occur when a person gets too hot, loses fluid by sweating, and doesn't consume enough fluids (dehydration).

- Observe the child for symptoms of heat exhaustion, including:
    » Weakness or dizziness
    » Nausea
    » Painful muscle spasms. *See section on Heat Cramps on the next page for more information.*
- Move the child to a cool place or cool the child's body with wet, cool cloths or pour cool water over his skin.
- Encourage the child to sip water.
- Observe the child for symptoms of **heat stroke** or **dehydration.** *See the Heat Stroke section below and the Dehydration section on the next page for more information.*

**CALL EMS (911) IF:**

- The child's body temperature rises. *See "FEVER" for more information on taking a child's temperature.*
- You observe any symptoms of heat stroke. *See the Heat Stroke section below for more information.*
- The child shows symptoms of shock. *See the section on Shock under "SUDDEN ILLNESS" for more information.*
- The child does not feel better in a few minutes.

## Heat Stroke

Heat stroke is life-threatening! The child's body temperature increases and can quickly reach 108°F or higher. The child must be cooled *quickly* to avoid permanent brain damage.

figure 12

**CALL EMS (911).**  This is a life-threatening emergency!

- Move the child to a cool place and cool the child's body fast!
- Remove unnecessary clothing from the child.
- Pour cool water over the child's head and body, or place the child in a tub of cool water. Avoid getting water in the child's nose or mouth.
- Place cloth-wrapped cold packs in the child's armpits and groin. *See figure 12.*

- If the child is awake, give him sips of cool water.
- If the child vomits, turn the child's head and body to the side to prevent choking.

**OBSERVE THE CHILD FOR SYMPTOMS OF HEAT STROKE, INCLUDING:**
- Hot, red, dry skin (no sweating)
- Elevated body temperature (fever). *See "FEVER" for more information on taking a child's temperature.*
- Rapid heartbeat
- Breathing problems (shortness of breath, wheezing, coughing)
- Headache
- Weakness, dizziness, fainting
- Confusion or decreasing level of responsiveness

## Heat Cramps

Heat cramps are brief, severe cramps in the leg, arm, or abdomen that can occur after playing in hot weather or a hot environment. They are painful but usually not serious.
- Move the child to a cool place.
- Encourage the child to drink water.
- Gently massage the painful area.
- Observe the child for symptoms of heat exhaustion, heat stroke, or dehydration.

## Dehydration

Dehydration occurs when a child doesn't drink enough water or fluid to replace fluid lost through perspiration, urination, diarrhea, or vomiting.
- Observe the child for symptoms of dehydration, including:
  » Dry skin and mouth
  » Sunken eyes
  » Failure to urinate within 6 daytime hours of last urination; urine is dark in color
  » Crying with few tears
- Encourage the child to drink liquids, including:
  » Water
  » Oral rehydration solutions such as Pedialyte
- **Do not** give milk, salty broths, fruit juices, or carbonated beverages.
- Call EMS (911). Dehydration can be very dangerous, especially for infants and young children.

### Sunburn

- Remove the child from sun exposure. Move the child to a cool place.
- Skin may be red and abnormally warm. The child may complain of pain.
- Apply cool compresses to relieve pain.
- Do not apply ointments or lotions (unless you have written authorization and lotion is prescribed specifically for that child).
- Observe the child for symptoms of heat-related illness.
  » Call EMS (911) if the child's body temperature is elevated (fever). This can indicate **heat stroke**, a life-threatening problem.
  » Encourage the child to sip water. Observe the child for signs of dehydration.
- Contact the child's family and recommend medical attention if:
  » An infant under one year of age is sunburned.
  » The sunburned skin includes blisters.
  » The child is in pain.
  » There is swelling related to the sunburn, especially around the eyes.

---

## PRₓESCRIPTION FOR PREVENTION

- Be aware of heat and UV index for outdoor play. Plan indoor, air-conditioned activities during the sunniest part of summer days.
- Avoid outdoor activities during the hottest part of the day (11:00–2:00). Provide a shaded area for children's play.
- Help children dress appropriately for warm weather. Removable layers are best.
- Provide water and encourage children to drink frequently throughout the day.
- Never leave children unattended in vehicles.
- Recommend that families provide sunscreen to prevent sunburn.

# Cold-Related Conditions

## Frostnip

Frostnip is a nonfreezing injury of the skin tissues, usually of the fingers, toes, ears, cheeks, and chin. It is the most common cold injury. Frostnip also can occur if ice or a cold pack is placed directly on a child's skin. Always wrap ice packs or cold packs in a soft cloth, or place a cloth or towel between the child's skin and the cold pack. Symptoms of frostnip include:

- Reddened, gray, or pale skin
- Stiff-feeling skin with soft and resilient underlying tissue. If a person presses against the tissue, the skin indentation springs back.
- Injured tissues that turn pink or even red as the body part is warmed
- The child indicates numbness or tingling as skin is warmed

If you suspect frostnip:

- Take the child to a warm place. If a warm place is not immediately available, place cold body parts close to warm body areas (tuck cold hands into armpits, for example).
- Allow cold-injured parts to *slowly* return to normal body temperature.
- **Do not** rub affected areas.
- Keep the child warm. Prevent refreezing of area, which could cause severe tissue damage.
- Contact the child's family and recommend they contact their physician for further instruction.

## Frostbite

Frostbite is tissue damage caused by freezing of the body tissue. The ears, face, hands, and feet are most likely to be affected.

- Call EMS (911).
- Observe the child for symptoms of frostbite, including:
  - » Injured skin appears pale or bluish.
  - » Skin and tissue may feel cold, solid, and woodlike. If a person presses against the tissue, the skin indentation **does not** spring back.
  - » The child indicates skin feels numb.
  - » Injured skin may have small blisters containing either clear or bloody fluid.
  - » As the body part is warmed, injured tissues may turn pink or red. If damage is severe, tissue may remain pale.
  - » Injured tissue may hurt, tingle, or feel like it is burning as it warms.

- Take the child to a warm place. If a warm place is not immediately available, place cold body parts close to warm body areas (for example, tuck cold hands into armpits).
- Remove wet clothes, shoes, and socks. Dress the child in clean, dry clothes or wrap her in a warm blanket while waiting for EMS to arrive.
- Allow cold-injured parts to *slowly* return to normal body temperature.
- Put frostbitten hands or feet into warm, not hot, water.
- Do not allow a child to walk on feet you suspect are frostbitten.
- **Do not** rub affected areas. **Do not** rub the area with snow.
- If fingers or toes are cold-damaged, put dry gauze between the fingers/toes.
- If blisters are present, cover with gauze. Do not break blisters.
- Contact the child's family after EMS (911) has been called.

## Hypothermia

Hypothermia occurs when the core body temperature drops below 95°F. Hypothermia is often caused by falling into cold water or being outside too long without protective clothing.

- Call EMS (911).
- Observe the child for symptoms of hypothermia, including:
  » A lower-than-normal body temperature
  » Confusion or unresponsiveness
  » Unconsciousness
- Warm the child quickly. Take the child to a warm place. If a warm place is not immediately available, hold the child close to someone else's warm body.
- Remove wet clothes, shoes, and socks. Dress the child in warm, dry clothes or wrap in a warm blanket.
- Keep the child wrapped in a blanket while waiting for first responders to arrive.
- Contact the child's family after EMS (911) has been called.

---

### PRₓESCRIPTION FOR PREVENTION

- Help children dress appropriately for cold weather. Removable layers are best.
- Limit children's time outside in very cold weather. If there is a combination of severe cold and wind chill, plan indoor activities.

# Convulsions and Seizures

**CALL EMS (911) IF:**

- The child has breathing difficulties (shortness of breath, wheezing, coughing).
- The child has no known seizure history.
- You do not have a seizure care plan for the child.
- The child remains unconscious or unresponsive after a seizure.
- The child falls or hits his head during a seizure.
- Contact the family after EMS (911) has been called.

**CONVULSIONS AND SEIZURES:**

- Gently place the child on the floor or ground.
- If the child is drooling or vomits, position the child on his side.
- Loosen tight-fitting clothing around head or neck.
- Remove nearby objects (such as furniture and toys).
- Protect the child's head from impact by sliding the palm of your hand, a towel, or a blanket under the child's head. *See figure 13.*
- **Do not** put your fingers or any object in the mouth of a child during a seizure.
- Observe the child for breathing. Perform CPR if necessary. *See "CPR" for more information.*

figure 13

- Document the time the seizure begins and ends.
  Provide a detailed description of the episode to the family and medical personnel. Notice which extremities are involved (one side, both sides, arm and/or leg, for example). Note if the child had a fever or acted ill before the seizure.
- After seizure has stopped, open airway if the child is not breathing—begin CPR. *See "CPR" for more information.*

# Sudden Illness

## Shock

Shock is a life-threatening condition that causes very low, inadequate blood pressure. Shock occurs because the body is not getting enough blood flow. It can occur as a reaction to illness, injury, bleeding, dehydration, or allergic reaction.

Call EMS (911). **Shock requires immediate medical treatment.** It can get worse rapidly.

**OBSERVE THE CHILD FOR SYMPTOMS OF SHOCK, INCLUDING:**
- Pale, cool, or clammy skin
- Weak, rapid pulse
- Shallow breathing
- Unresponsiveness or unconsciousness
- If the child is conscious, he or she may feel faint, very weak, or confused.

**TREATMENT AND PREVENTION OF SHOCK INCLUDE:**
- Calming the child
- Keeping the child warm (not hot) and as comfortable as possible. Loosen tight clothing.
- Having the child lie down on her back with feet higher than the head. However, if raising the legs could cause pain or further injury, keep the child flat.
- Observing the child for breathing problems

## Fainting

Fainting is a sudden and temporary loss of responsiveness caused by a brief lack of adequate blood and oxygen to the brain.
- Evaluate the situation and determine a possible cause for the fainting, such as:
  » The child has not eaten sufficiently.
  » The child reacted to a situation (stress, fear of needles, or sight of blood, for example).
  » The child reacted to pain.
  » The child overexerted herself physically or became too hot.
  » The child has been standing too long.
  » The child was holding her breath during a crying episode.
  » Heat stroke
  » Bleeding

- Lay the child on her back to prevent falling.
- Elevate the legs 8 to 12 inches.
- Loosen tight-fitting clothing.
- Observe the child for breathing difficulties (shortness of breath, wheezing, coughing). Perform CPR if necessary. *See "CPR" for more information.*

**CALL EMS (911) IF:**
- The child remains unresponsive for more than a **minute or so**.
- The child fell while fainting and possibly received a blow to the head.
- The child becomes blue or pale.
- Fainting is associated with:
    » An injury, particularly a head injury
    » Illness or fever
    » Pain
    » Allergic reaction

## Asthma or Chronic Respiratory Condition

If a child has been diagnosed with asthma or other chronic respiratory condition:
- Staff should work with the child's family and health care professionals to develop an emergency care plan or asthma action plan.
- Any prescribed medications or supplies (such as peak flow meters, quick-acting inhalers, spacers, or epinephrine auto-injectors) must be kept near the child at all times. Medications must be properly stored and out of children's reach.
- Teachers directly involved in the care of the child should have specific training related to the child's condition, including how to manage an acute asthma attack (or other respiratory-related emergency) and how to administer medications.
- Other staff members involved in the care of the child should be aware of the condition and that there is an emergency care plan.
- Some state laws allow licensed child care providers to administer inhaled medication for respiratory problems such as asthma. Check your local licensing regulations and follow procedures established by signed parental medical authorization.

**IN CASE OF AN ASTHMA EPISODE OR OTHER RESPIRATORY DISTRESS:**
- Follow the child's emergency care plan or asthma action plan.
- Use a quick-acting inhaled medication only if it has been prescribed for that child.
- Observe the child's breathing. If normal breathing does not resume within 10 minutes, follow the emergency care plan, including calling EMS (911).
- If the child is not breathing, begin CPR.

## Diabetic Reaction/Hypoglycemia

**IF A CHILD IS DIAGNOSED WITH DIABETES OR ANOTHER CHRONIC CONDITION:**

- Teachers should work with the child's health care professionals to develop an emergency care plan.
- Any prescribed medications or supplies (such as glucose monitors or insulin) must be kept near the child at all times. Medications must be properly stored and out of children's reach.
- Teachers directly involved in the care of the child must have specific training related to the child's condition, including administration of medication and emergency care.
- Other staff members involved in the care of the child should be aware of the condition and that there is an emergency care plan.
- Maintain written authorization forms of when and how to check the child's blood sugar levels.

**Hypoglycemia** (low blood sugar level) is one of the most frequent complications of diabetes. It can happen suddenly. Most hypoglycemic episodes are mild.

Symptoms may include the following:

- Headache
- Shakiness or tremors
- Dizziness
- Increased heart rate or palpitations
- Pale skin
- Clammy skin or sweating
- Lethargy
- Changing level of responsiveness, including mood changes

Treatment for hypoglycemia:

- Have the child eat or drink fast-acting carbohydrates, such as fruit juice, fruit beverage, crackers, or other food as indicated in the child's emergency care plan.
- Follow the child's emergency care plan, including contacting the child's family or EMS (911) if indicated.

## Abdominal Pain

Mild abdominal pain may be due to a number of causes, including overeating and intestinal gas. Severe abdominal pain, or pain accompanied by other symptoms, may indicate serious illness or injury.

- Contact the child's family and recommend immediate medical attention if you observe or the child complains of these symptoms:
    - » Severe abdominal pain
    - » Localized pain (such as pain on one side)
    - » Pain accompanied by vomiting or fever
    - » Bloody stools (bowel movement)
    - » Pain after a fall or blow to the abdomen
- **Do not** give the child anything to eat or drink.
- Testicular (scrotal) pain is often described by young boys as abdominal pain.
    - » Scrotal pain is a medical emergency.
    - » Contact the child's family and recommend medical attention.

## Other Symptoms That May Indicate Illness or Injury

If you observe or the child complains of these or other symptoms, contact the child's family and recommend medical attention.

- Unexplained pain
- Stiffness of the neck
- Vomiting and/or diarrhea, especially in combination with fever or other symptoms
- Lethargy, listlessness
- Sudden onset of rash
- Unexplainable confusion
- Looking or acting severely ill
- Unexpected behavior or mood swings

### PRESCRIPTION FOR PREVENTION

- Young children do not always respond to pain or discomfort as expected. A child may have a serious injury, such as a broken bone, and not complain or show pain or discomfort.
- Know the children in your care. If you think a child has an illness or injury, even if there are no obvious symptoms, contact the child's family. As appropriate, recommend or arrange for a child's health care. Follow your intuition!

# Fever

Fever is a body temperature that is higher than normal. The average normal body temperature is 98.6°F. A child can develop a high fever very quickly.

- Observe the child for symptoms of fever, including:
  - » A flushed face
  - » Hot skin that may be either dry or sweaty
  - » Body (forehead, abdomen, back) feels hot
- Evaluate the situation and determine a possible cause for the fever, such as:
  - » The child (especially an infant) is dressed or covered too warmly. Remove unnecessary blankets and/or clothing.
  - » The environment is too warm (children playing outside in warm weather, for example). Move the child to a cooler environment. Observe the child for symptoms of heat exhaustion or heat stroke. *See "HEAT-RELATED CONDITIONS" for more information.*
  - » A recent immunization. A fever may occur within the first 24 to 48 hours.
  - » An illness or infection. Observe the child for additional symptoms of illness or injury.
- Take the child's temperature. *See the section on Taking a Child's Temperature on the following pages for more information.*
  - » Recorded body temperature may vary depending on how the temperature is taken.
- If thermometer reading indicates normal body temperature (98.6°F):
  - » Continue to observe the child for symptoms of fever or other illness or injury.
  - » Continue to evaluate the environment and eliminate cause of overheating (child overdressed, room too hot, child playing outdoors on hot day).
  - » Prevent dehydration. Offer infants breast milk or formula. Offer water to older children. *See "HEAT-RELATED CONDITIONS" for more information on dehydration.*
  - » If symptoms persist, contact the child's family.

## Response to Elevated Body Temperature (fever)

(NOTE: Normal body temperature is 98.6°F if measured with an ear thermometer. Axillary [under the arm] temperature is approximately 97.6°F—or 1 degree less than normal body temperature.) *See the section on Taking a Child's Temperature on the following pages for more information.*

- Young infant (age 3 months or younger):
  - » Any fever (such as an axillary temperature over 99°F) indicates a need for medical attention.
  - » Contact the child's family and recommend immediate medical attention.

- Infant (age 4 to 12 months) and older:
  - » Oral, forehead, or ear temperature of 102°F or higher (or axillary temperature of 103°F or higher) indicates a need for medical attention.
  - » Contact the child's family and recommend medical attention.
- **Do not** give medication to lower temperature.

Fever is not a disease; it is a symptom. Fever accompanied by other symptoms may indicate a serious or life-threatening condition.

**CALL EMS (911) IF FEVER IS ACCOMPANIED BY OTHER SYMPTOMS, INCLUDING:**
- Fainting, seizure, or convulsions
- Stiff neck
- Irregular breathing
- Symptoms of heat stroke *See "HEAT-RELATED CONDITIONS" for more information.*

**CONTACT THE CHILD'S** family and recommend medical attention if fever is accompanied by other symptoms, including:
- Fussiness, changing level of responsiveness, or unusual sleepiness
- Not eating or drinking adequately to stay hydrated
- Confusion
- Rash
- Ear pain (child is tugging on his ear)
- Persistent sore throat
- Vomiting and/or diarrhea
- Painful, burning, or frequent urination

## Taking a Child's Temperature

Caregivers should be trained in the proper use of a thermometer.
- Electronic ear thermometers (also called tympanic or aural thermometers):
  - » These are quick, accurate, and easy to use.
  - » Always use a disposable thermometer cover.
  - » Follow manufacturer's instructions for your specific thermometer. Store the instruction sheet with the thermometer.
  - » Ear thermometers are not recommended for young infants (age 3 months or less) because the infant's ear canal is so small. Use an axillary (under arm) temperature-taking method for very young infants.
- Temporal artery thermometers:
  - » These electronic thermometers, which are rubbed gently across the temple and forehead, are quick, accurate, easy to use, and noninvasive.
  - » Can be easily cleaned with alcohol between uses.
  - » Follow manufacturer's instructions for your specific thermometer. Store the instruction sheet with the thermometer.

- Plastic digital thermometers:
  » These inexpensive thermometers are quick, accurate, and easy to use.
  » Always use a disposable thermometer cover.
  » Response time varies, so it's best to select one that beeps when the child's temperature is recorded.
  » Follow manufacturer's instructions for your specific thermometer. Store the instruction sheet with the thermometer.
  » These can be used to measure temperature either axillary (under the arm) or oral (in the mouth).
- **Never** use a glass thermometer.

Caregivers should use noninvasive methods to measure a child's body temperature. Only trained caregivers should be allowed to take a child's temperature.

### DIGITAL THERMOMETER
- Choose a digital thermometer. Make sure the digital thermometer is in the "ON" mode.
- Dry the child's armpit with a soft cloth.
- Place the thermometer in the child's armpit. Gently hold the arm down close to the child's body. *See figure 14.*
- Hold the child in this position until the digital thermometer beeps.
- Read the thermometer. Normal axillary temperature is 97.6°F (1 degree *less* than the normal body temperature of 98.6°F).

### EAR THERMOMETER
- An ear thermometer is recommended for infants age 4 months and older, and for children.
- Follow manufacturer's instructions for use.

*figure 14*

### OTHER CONSIDERATIONS
- **Do not** take a child's temperature rectally (in the bottom).
- Oral (mouth) temperature recordings are **not** recommended. The accuracy can be affected by the placement in the child's mouth, opening or breathing through the mouth, or if the child has eaten or drunk something hot or cold. Oral temperature should not be used for infants.
- **Never** use a glass thermometer.
- Use a disposable thermometer cover.

# Dental Injuries

### Injury to the Lip, Tongue, or Gums

- Put on non-latex gloves.
- Help the child sit up with head tilted slightly forward, or lie on one side to prevent blood from going down the airway.
- Help the child rinse her mouth with water so you can identify the injured area.
- Apply direct pressure to the bleeding area with gauze or a clean cloth.
- Apply cold compresses to reduce swelling.
- Contact the child's family and recommend immediate dental or medical care.

### CALL EMS (911) IF:

- Bleeding does not stop after 5 minutes of continuous direct pressure.
- The wound is deep or large.
- The wound cuts across the tongue.
- The wound involves the back or roof of the mouth or the throat.
- The wound involves the lip and face.
- The wound is from an animal bite.

### Broken Tooth

- Put on non-latex gloves.
- Help the child rinse her mouth with water so you can identify the injured area.
- Give the child a cold compress to hold on the injured tooth, or hold a cold compress on her face in the area of the broken tooth.
- Collect all the pieces of the tooth. Put pieces in a tooth preservation kit (such as Save-A-Tooth or EMT ToothSaver [see First Aid Supplies]), or in a cold, wet cloth or in a container (such as a plastic zipper bag) of milk.
- Call the child's family to arrange for immediate dental care.

### Knocked-Out Tooth

- Put on non-latex gloves.
- Position the child to prevent blood from going down the airway. Help the child sit up with head tilted slightly forward, or lie on one side.
- Help the child rinse her mouth with water so you can identify the injured area.
- If bleeding, apply direct pressure to the area with gauze or a clean cloth.
- Give the child a cold compress to hold on the injured area, or hold a cold compress on her face in the area of the knocked-out tooth.

- Attempt to find the tooth. If you find the tooth:
  - » Hold the tooth by the crown (the top), not the root.
  - » Remove visible dirt by gently rinsing with water. Do not scrub the tooth.
- Keep the tooth moist.
  - » If there is concern that the child might swallow the tooth if you try to replace it, put the tooth in a preservation kit (such as Save-A-Tooth or EMT ToothSaver [see First Aid Supplies]), or in a cold, wet cloth or a container of milk.
  - » For an older child, and if the child can cooperate, replace the tooth gently in the socket, then have the child bite down on a gauze pad or cloth to keep it in place.
- Contact the child's family and arrange for *immediate* dental care. Professional dental care within 1 to 2 hours may save the tooth.
- Professional dental care is important, even if the knocked-out tooth cannot be found.

## Toothache

A toothache may be a dental emergency (an abscessed or injured tooth, for example), or it may refer to more common discomfort associated with teething, mouth sores, earache or ear infection, or sinus infection. Toothaches may also be caused by food caught between the teeth.

- Put on non-latex gloves.
- Help the child rinse her mouth with water.
- If the child's toothbrush (or a new, clean toothbrush) is available, have the child brush her teeth thoroughly.
- If the child can cooperate, floss her teeth gently to remove any food that might be lodged between teeth.
  - » Break off about 18 inches of floss and wind most of it around one of your middle fingers. Wind the remaining floss around the same finger of the opposite hand. Hold the floss tightly between your thumbs and forefingers.
  - » Guide the floss between the teeth using a gentle rubbing motion.
  - » When the floss reaches the gum line, curve it into a C-shape against one tooth. Gently slide it into the space between the gum and the tooth.
  - » Hold the floss tightly against the tooth. Gently rub the side of the tooth, moving the floss away from the gum with back and forth motions.
- Again, help the child rinse her mouth with water. Removal of lodged food may alleviate the pain.

**IF THE CHILD STILL COMPLAINS OF PAIN:**

- Give the child a cold compress to hold on her face in the area of the toothache.
- Contact the child's family and recommend dental or medical care.
- Recommend immediate dental or medical care if:
  » The pain is very severe.
  » The child has a fever.
  » The child's face is swollen.
  » The child is acting very sick.

## PRESCRIPTION FOR PREVENTION

- Keep pathways and children's play areas clear of debris to prevent falls.
- Keep supplies on hand for emergency tooth preservations. Two such products available are Save-A-Tooth and the EMT ToothSaver.

# Eye, Ear, and Nose Emergencies

## Eye Trauma

Eye trauma refers to any injury to the eye. Eye injury is the most common and preventable cause of blindness. Immediate medical attention is needed for any eye injury.

- Call EMS (911) for any injury to the eye or the eye area.
- Call EMS (911) if you observe or the child complains of any of the following symptoms related to the eye or vision:
  » Blood in the eye
  » Inability to open the eye after trauma
  » Pain when moving the eye
  » Redness and swelling of the eyelid
  » Extreme sensitivity to light
  » Double vision
  » Decrease in vision
  » Numbness in the eye

## Chemical Injury to Eye

- Put on non-latex gloves.
- Immediately rinse the injured eye with water.
  » Have the child lie on one side (same side as injured eye). Place a towel under the child's head (to absorb water).
  » Hold the injured eye open. You may need assistance for this.
  » Using a cup or small pitcher, pour cool water over the injured eye. Flush with water so that water flows from the inside corner (by nose) toward the outside corner of the eye (toward the ear). *See figure 15.*
- Call EMS (911).
- Call the Poison Control Center at 800-222-1222.
- Continue rinsing the eye until first responders arrive and are able to take over.

*figure 15*

### Scratch, Cut, or Penetrating Injury to Eye or Eye Area

- Call EMS (911).
- Put on non-latex gloves.
- Keep the child as quiet as possible. It is best for the child to lie still, flat on his back, but do not force the child to lie down.
- If the child will cooperate, attempt to cover the eye with an eye shield or paper cup. This will help protect the eye. If possible, cover both eyes to reduce movement of the eyeball.
- **Do not** apply any pressure to the eye.

### Foreign Object in Eye (dust, sand)

- Put on non-latex gloves.
- Check for dust, sand, or another object in the eye if you observe or the child complains of any of the following symptoms:
  - » Rubbing the eye
  - » Watery or reddened eye
  - » Itching or scratchy feeling
  - » Pain
  - » Sensitivity to light
  - » Blurry vision

figure 16

- Keep the child from pressing on or rubbing the eye.
- Gently examine the eye. *See figure 16.*
  - » Pull the lower lid down and ask the child to look up.
  - » Then hold the upper lid while the child looks down.
- If the object is obviously floating (moving) in the tear film on the surface of the eye, try flushing it out.
  - » Have the child lie on one side (same side as injured eye). Place a towel under the child's head (to absorb water).
  - » Hold the injured eye open. You may need assistance for this.
  - » Using a cup or small pitcher, pour cool water over the injured eye. Flush with water so that water flows from the inside corner (by nose) toward the outside corner of the eye (toward the ear).
- **Do not** try to remove an object except by flushing with water.
- **Do not** attempt to touch the object.
- Contact the child's family and recommend immediate medical attention (preferably an ophthalmologist or primary care physician) if:
  - » The object is not easily flushed out.
  - » The object appears to be embedded in the eye.
  - » The child continues to complain of pain, irritation, or blurred vision.
  - » The eye continues to be red or swelling is present.

## Blunt Force Trauma to Eye or Eye Area (black eye)

- Gently apply cold compresses intermittently: 5 to 10 minutes on, 10 to 15 minutes off.
- Contact the child's family and recommend medical evaluation. Blunt force trauma (such as getting hit by a ball or a fist) can cause internal damage.

**CALL EMS (911) IF ANY OF THE FOLLOWING SYMPTOMS ARE OBSERVED:**

- Drainage from the eye
- Any visible abnormality of the eyeball
- Visible bleeding on the white part of the eye

Contact the child's family and recommend *immediate* medical attention (preferably an ophthalmologist) if any of the following symptoms are observed:

- Increased redness
- Persistent eye pain
- Any changes in vision

## Other Symptoms Related to Eyes and Vision

Contact the child's family and recommend medical attention if you observe or the child complains of any of the following symptoms:

- Redness, or "bloodshot" eyes
- Excessive rubbing of the eyes, itching, or irritation
- Discharge or "crusty" particles, especially after the child has been asleep
- Squinting or holding objects close to the face when playing

---

### PRₓESCRIPTION FOR PREVENTION

- Teach children to avoid throwing sand and dirt into the air.
- Keep all spray and aerosol substances out of children's reach.

---

## Earache

Pain in or around the ear area may be caused by a variety of conditions, including ear infection, teething, sinus infection, or other illness or injury.

- Symptoms of ear pain may include crying, fever, and fussiness—especially if the child is also pulling or rubbing his ear.
- Contact the child's family and arrange for medical attention.

## Foreign Object in Ear

A foreign object (such as a rock, insect, or bean) in the ear canal can cause pain and hearing loss.

- Using a flashlight or other bright light, look inside the child's ear canal.
- If the object is clearly visible, is flexible, and can be grasped easily with tweezers, gently remove it.
- If the object cannot be grasped with tweezers, tilt the child's head to the affected side and keep the child still. Contact the child's family and arrange for medical attention.
- **Do not** probe the ear with a cotton swab, matchstick, or other tool. This could push the object farther into the ear.

Contact the child's family and recommend medical attention if:

- The object cannot easily be removed.
- The child continues to complain of pain after the object is removed.
- There is bleeding in the ear.
- The ear continues to be red or swelling is present.
- The child appears to have hearing loss.

## Foreign Object in Nose

Children sometimes insert objects, such as a rock or bean, in their noses.

- Contact the child's family and recommend medical attention.

# Resources

American Academy of Pediatrics, *Healthy Child Care America,* www.healthychildcare.org.

American Academy of Pediatrics. *Pediatric First Aid for Caregivers and Teachers*. (Pedfacts) www.pedfactsonline.com.

American Academy of Pediatrics, American Public Health Association, and National Resource Center for Health and Safety in Child Care and Early Education. *Caring for Our Children: National Health and Safety Performance Standards: Guidelines for Out-of-Home Child Care Programs*. 3rd ed. Elk Grove Village, IL: American Academy of Pediatrics, and Washington, DC: American Public Health Association, 2011. www.nrckids.org.

American Heart Association. www.americanheart.org.

American Red Cross. www.redcross.org

Aronson, Susan S., and Timothy R. Shope, eds. *Managing Infectious Diseases in Child Care and Schools: A Quick Reference Guide*. 3rd ed. Elk Grove Village, IL: American Academy of Pediatrics, 2013.

Hendricks, Charlotte M. *Hip on Health: Health Information for Caregivers and Families*. St. Paul, MN: Redleaf Press, 2014.

Hendricks, Charlotte M., and Michele B. Pettibone. *Disaster Planning and Preparedness in Early Childhood and Schoolage Care Settings*. St. Paul, MN: Redleaf Press, 2014.

Mayo Clinic. *Choking: First Aid*. www.mayoclinic.org/first-aid/first-aid-choking/basics/art-20056637.

National Program for Playground Safety, www.playgroundsafety.org.

National Resource Center for Health and Safety in Child Care and Early Education, *Individual States' Child Care Licensure Regulations,* nrckids.org/index.cfm/resources/state-licensing-and-regulation-information.

Smith, Connie Jo, Charlotte M. Hendricks, and Becky S. Bennett. *Growing, Growing Strong: A Whole Health Curriculum for Young Children*. St. Paul, MN: Redleaf Press, 2014.

U.S. Consumer Product Safety Commission. *Handbook for Public Playground Safety*. Washington, DC: U.S. Consumer Product Safety Commission, 2010. Available for download at www.cpsc.gov/CPSCPUB/PUBS/325.pdf.

# Credits

## Author

DR. CHARLOTTE M. HENDRICKS, PhD, founder and president of www.childhealthonline.org, has been promoting health education for young children, families, and teachers for over thirty years. She provides training sessions for Head Start and early childhood programs, presents at state and national conferences, develops curricula and training modules, and writes books. Her other Redleaf Press books include the Growing, Growing Strong series, *Hip on Health*, and *Disaster Planning and Preparedness in Early Childhood and Schoolage Care Settings*.

## Medical Reviewers

Elaine Abrams, RN, CHES, MPH
Community Health Coordinator
Nursing & Home Care
Wilton, CT

Dianne Steudel Burdette, RN, BSN, CPN
Child Care Health Consultant Coordinator
The Children's Home Society of New Jersey

Brenda Davis, RN
Childcare Nurse Consultant
Healthy Childcare Alabama

Cyndy Henderson, RN, MSN
Childcare Nurse Consultant
Healthy Childcare Alabama

Kathy Hunt, RDH
Healthy Smiles Community
Dental Hygiene Program
Wamego, KS

Sharis LeMay, RN, BNCSN
Assistant Director of Children's Health
Alabama Dept. of Public Health

Marie Mitchell
Health Information Specialist
Pembroke, KY

Bryan A. Nelson*, MD
Hennepin County Medical Center
Minneapolis, MN

Donald Palmer*, MD
Fairhope, AL

Debbie Parker, RN, BSN
Childcare Nurse Consultant
Healthy Childcare Alabama

Daphne Pate, RN
Childcare Nurse Consultant
Healthy Childcare Alabama

Wayne Schneider*, EMT-P
First Response Training, Inc.
Eden Prairie, MN

Jennifer A. Schmitz*, PA-C
Hennepin County Medical Center
Minneapolis, MN

Hilary Pert Stecklein, MD
St. Paul, MN

* Reviewer for revised edition.